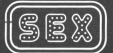

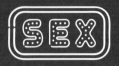

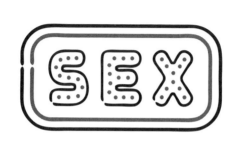

SEX: 369 FACTS TO BLOW YOU AWAY

Summersdale Publishers Ltd
46 West Street
Chichester
West Sussex
PO19 1RP
UK

www.summersdale.com

Printed and bound in the Czech Republic

ISBN: 978-1-84953-501-4

Substantial discounts on bulk quantities of Summersdale books are available to corporations, professional associations and other organisations. For details contact Nicky Douglas by telephone: +44 (0) 1243 756902, fax: +44 (0) 1243 786300 or email: nicky@summersdale.com.

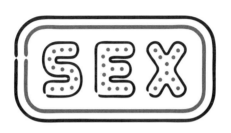

SEX

369 FACTS
TO BLOW
YOU AWAY

SADIE CAYMAN

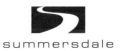

summersdale

① There are at least 100 million acts of sexual intercourse each day. In other words, around 65,000 couples are having sex at this moment around the world.

② Typically a person spends about 600 hours having sex between the age of 20 and 70.

③ Anorgasmia is a sexual dysfunction whose sufferers cannot experience an orgasm.

(4) Researchers from the University of California found that men who helped with the housework got 50 per cent more sex than those who did none.

(5) Agalmatophilia is a sexual attraction to statues or mannequins.

(6) The word 'sex' was coined in the fourteenth century, from the Latin *sexus*.

(7) Reports claim that the highest number of orgasms experienced by a woman in an hour is 134; by a man, 16.

(8) In America, 80 per cent of men have been circumcised, compared to less than 20 per cent of their counterparts in the UK.

(9) Complete sexual inactivity may lead to a reduction in penis size.

HALF AN HOUR OF SEX IS SAID TO BURN BETWEEN 85 AND 200 CALORIES, THOUGH IT DEPENDS ON THE LEVEL OF ACTIVITY INVOLVED. (200 CALORIES IS EQUIVALENT TO 15 MINUTES ON A TREADMILL.)

(11) Russian woman Tatyana Kozhevnikova is reported to be the world-record holder for lifting the most weights – 14 kg – with her vaginal muscles.

(12) Sex makes you feel less tired as it releases endorphins that boost energy.

(13) The proteins in sperm give it anti-wrinkle properties when rubbed into the skin.

(14) Some modern languages have beautifully descriptive words for *dildo*, such as фаллоимитатор (Russian for 'phallic imitator'), *consolador* (Spanish for 'consoler'), and *cala goeg* (Welsh for 'fake penis').

(15) Spending time in the sun increases levels of vitamin D. For men, this boosts the sex hormone testosterone and therefore increases libido.

16 The Romans had three different words for types of kisses: *osculum* – a kiss on the cheek; *basium* – a kiss on the lips; *savolium* – a deep kiss.

17 Kissing may have been brought to Europe when Alexander the Great of Greece invaded India in *c.*326 BC.

18 Male llamas have sharp 'fighting teeth', used to bite off other males' testicles.

19 | A woman's lips are a visible expression of her fertility and health; the higher her oestrogen levels, the fuller her lips – making her more sexually attractive to men.

20 | Eunuchs in imperial China often rose to many of the top positions in society. They symbolised their rise to the upper ranks by keeping their genitals in a jar on a high shelf.

21 Lara Croft of the *Tomb Raider* series is regularly voted the sexiest female video game character. Samus Aran of *Metroid*, Rayne of *BloodRayne* and Joanna Dark of *Perfect Dark* all feature regularly on top ten lists.

22 Aerobic exercise that increases blood flow to the genital region, such as jogging, cycling or vigorous walking, will increase your libido.

23 Oculolinctus is the act of licking someone's eyeball for sexual pleasure.

24 'Cat-heads' is a slang expression, believed to have been coined in the nineteenth century, for a woman's breasts.

25 Of all nations, the Greeks claim to have the most sex (87 per cent say they have sex once a week).

26 Male and female emperor penguins stand facing each other for several minutes and appear to bow to each other before intercourse.

27 Emperor penguins stay faithful to one mate each year, but change partners from year to year – probably because of the chances of finding the same mate within the short breeding season are very low, after walking between 50 and 120 km to the colony's nesting areas.

28 Forty per cent of American college students say they know someone who has had sex with a professor or teaching assistant.

29 According to studies, most women climax easily through masturbation but sometimes struggle when with their partners; partly because of overactive minds thinking of other things, partly because of lack of foreplay.

30 Some women are allergic to semen – leading to itching and burning sensations.

31 Durex, the condom manufacturer, has invented an app that sends signals to small vibrators in your lover's underwear.

32 Men who smoke have twice the risk of developing erectile dysfunction as non-smokers; the link is strongest in younger men.

33 Smoking can affect testosterone levels, sperm count and sperm motility.

34 American writer Philip Roth caused scandal and controversy in 1969 when he published *Portnoy's Complaint*, about a sex-obsessed, sexually frustrated teenager who masturbates using various props, including a piece of liver.

FORMICOPHILIA IS A SEXUAL PLEASURE DERIVED FROM THE FEELING OF SMALL INSECTS CRAWLING OVER THE SKIN AND/ OR STINGING/BITING THE PRIVATE PARTS.

36 The sea slug is a 'simultaneous
    hermaphrodite', able to
    use its penis and vagina
    at the same time.

37 A type of Pacific coral reef sea
    slug has a penis equipped
    with spines. It can shed these
    after intercourse but they
    grow back the next day.

38 Women make more noise
    than men during sex.

39 Pheromones are chemicals released by our bodies. Some of these have the function of arousing potential partners when they're detected.

40 The *Literary Review*'s Bad Sex in Fiction award was established 'to draw attention to the crude and often perfunctory use of redundant passages of sexual description in the modern novel – and to discourage it'.

41 *La petite mort*, or 'the little death', is a French expression used to describe the moment of physical and spiritual release just after orgasm.

42 The testicles of a species of bush-cricket, or katydid, are larger than its head and account for up to 14 per cent of its body weight, the equivalent of a male human having testicles weighing 5 kg; this allows it to mate with many different females.

43) Colourful, flamboyant tropical fish have poorer quality sperm than their less attractive counterparts.

44) The ostracod, a millimetre-long sea creature, produces giant sperm up to ten times longer than its body.

45) The US state of Minnesota specifies that it is illegal for a man to have sex with a live fish; it says nothing about dead fish.

46 Approximately one in every 50 women has an extra nipple.

47 Each year around 11,000 Americans are injured when attempting unusual sexual positions.

48 During the Victorian age, when public standards of morality were extremely strict, there were up to 80,000 prostitutes working in London.

49 Prostitution is legal in most countries, including Iran, where 'temporary wives' can be obtained for a few hours, though it's a crime to advocate it, or aid or abet a woman to enter prostitution or operate a brothel – punishable by execution.

50 Wearing two condoms does not give extra protection against leaking; it actually raises the chances of breakage due to friction.

51 A study found that only 28.6 per cent of women always have an orgasm during intercourse with their partner.

52 Although it sounds risqué, the Condom Casino Tour is a programme that visits American universities to educate students about safe sex, through games such as Beer Goggle Black Jack and STD Bingo.

53 Twelve per cent of American women in a survey said they would have sex with a president if propositioned.

54 Low levels of oestrogen, which occur during the menopause, can leave the vagina too dry for comfortable sex.

55 A 2004 survey by *ABC News* revealed that cheating on a partner is the most common sexual fantasy for Americans.

(56) The oldest known evidence of condom use is a cave painting in Grotte des Combarelles in France, estimated to be 12,000–15,000 years old.

(57) Authors in the *Proceedings of the National Academy of Sciences* claim that torso shape is the most important factor determining how attractive women find a man's body, followed by the size of his flaccid penis and his height.

58 In primate species where males compete with other males, the mating call made by the female attracts males and also gives information about her status and reproductive state.

59 The average time a person spends kissing in their lifetime is 20,160 minutes, or two weeks.

60 Good sex relieves stress and headaches by releasing pain-killing endorphins.

61 One testicle hangs a little lower than the other so they don't strike each other when a man is moving.

62 When a man sees a woman he finds attractive, he holds her gaze for approximately 8.2 seconds.

63 A condom kept in a wallet for a long time can deteriorate due to friction.

64   The human penis is much longer, compared to body size, than that of other primates such as bonobos, gorillas and orang-utans. The fact that humans interact standing face to face also makes the penis more obvious.

65   Sex is a natural beauty treatment for women as it helps produce oestrogen, which makes the hair shiny and the skin glow.

66 In Florida it was once illegal to have sexual relations with a porcupine. It's still not a good idea.

67 According to sexologist Serenella Salomoni, when married couples remove the television from their bedroom, the frequency of sex doubles.

68 According to a 2012 survey, 60 per cent of Britons prefer to have sex with the light off.

(69) The word 'masturbate' comes from the Latin *manus*, hand, and *stuprare*, to soil or make dirty. Despite its bad name, we now know that masturbation is actually good for you.

(70) The sale of sex toys, including vibrators, is banned in the US states of Mississippi and Alabama.

71

A 2009 SURVEY SHOWED
THAT 36 PER CENT OF
PEOPLE UNDER THE AGE
OF 35 GO ON FACEBOOK
AFTER HAVING SEX.

72 According to *Runner's World* magazine, two out of three runners say they fantasise about sex while running.

73 One out of 11 runners fantasise about running while having sex.

74 'Falsies', or bra padding, designed to make the breasts look bigger or more pointed, became popular during the 1950s.

75 Eating ginger stimulates the feelings of excitement associated with sex. It elevates your heart rate, gets your blood flowing and makes you excited for the night ahead.

76 The vibrator was first widely used in the Victorian era as a cure for 'hysteria'.

77 In several US states, condoms can only be sold by doctors.

(78) The fig leaf is associated with modesty, as in the biblical *Book of Genesis*, Adam and Eve used fig leaves to cover their nakedness after eating from the tree of knowledge.

(79) A plaster cast fig leaf was kept in the Victoria and Albert Museum during Queen Victoria's reign, to cover up the genitals of the plaster cast statue of Michelangelo's *David* when the queen or other female dignitary visited.

(80) In 2013, ancient Greek statues of nude male figures caused shock when displayed in Qatar as part of an Olympic Games exhibition. They were covered with veils, then returned to Greece.

(81) The sado-masochistic novel *Venus in Furs*, first published in 1870, has been adapted for film five times, as well as giving its name to a Velvet Underground album.

82 The sex icon Marilyn Monroe had problems reaching orgasm – she told a friend that she had never had an orgasm with any of her three husbands or various lovers.

83 A 'merkin' is a pubic wig; the word was first used in 1617. They were originally used by prostitutes in the fifteenth century who had shaved their pubic hair to combat lice, or to cover up signs of disease.

84 In Stanley Kubrick's 1964 anti-war black comedy film *Dr Strangelove*, the President of America is named Merkin Muffley.

85 Merkins are now used as erotic or decorative items, and in Hollywood films, to avoid full-frontal nudity.

86 A quarter of all penises are slightly bent when erect.

87 Peyronie's disease is a condition in which a man's penis has a painfully abnormal curve when erect.

88 In the animal world, only dolphins and bonobos are believed to have sex for pleasure, i.e. non-reproductive reasons.

89 There are seven calories in a teaspoon of semen.

90 It's more difficult to lie to someone you find sexually attractive.

91 Eating a lot of white bread and other refined carbohydrates (rather than wholegrain) can be bad for a man's sex drive, reducing energy and testosterone levels.

92   For every 16 kg an overweight man loses, his penis appears one inch longer.

93   In America, most couples over 65 still have sex at least once a week.

94   Viagra sales earned the pharmaceutical company Pfizer $2 billion in revenue in 2012.

(95) Seventy-three per cent of
men aged 70 are still potent.

(96) The most successful X-rated
movie of all time is *Deep Throat*.

(97) Victorian women wore
underwear with the crotch
area open and exposed for
hygiene reasons; contrary to
popular belief, Parisian cancan
dancers advanced the trend
for closed-crotch knickers.

98 Former porn star Annabel Chong, born Grace Quek in Singapore, was filmed engaging in 251 sex acts with 70 men over a period of ten hours, in January 1995 at the age of 22. She had advertised on television for men to participate in *The World's Biggest Gang Bang* as a way of challenging the notion of women as passive during sex.

99 Although testosterone is commonly thought of as a male sex hormone, women also need it for libido.

(100) The iron in a juicy steak helps blood flow and energy, and so can be good for libido. Red meat also has amino acids important for good mood, and zinc, important for production of testosterone. (Zinc is also found in beans, nuts and oysters.)

(101) In an American study in 2011, female respondents reported that they think about sex between one and 140 times a day.

102 Extra weight around the waist reduces the amount of a protein called SHBG (sex hormone-binding globulin) being produced in the liver, vital for testosterone.

103 Losing weight (more than 10 per cent of your body weight) too quickly causes sexual interest and enjoyment to fall.

104 The average speed of male ejaculation is 28 mph.

Once sperm enter the vagina, it takes them five minutes to travel six inches up the cervix.

 It takes sperm 72 hours to penetrate an egg.

 Seventy-five per cent of men always reach orgasm when making love.

108

GOING FOR A RUN GETS RID OF STRESSORS SUCH AS PENT-UP ENERGY, TENSION AND EXCESS ADRENALINE, WHILE RELEASING FEEL-GOOD ENDORPHINS, THEREFORE INCREASING SEX DRIVE.

109 In a *Glamour* magazine survey, 75 per cent of readers said they fantasised about their man dressing up as a fireman.

110 The first couple to be shown in bed together in an animated series in America were Fred and Wilma Flintstone in *The Flintstones*.

111 More women reach orgasm through clitoral stimulation than vaginal.

(112) The eighteenth-century Venetian adventurer Casanova wrote about his powers of seduction and affairs in *The Story of My Life*, earning him the reputation as the world's greatest lover – and womaniser.

(113) Men take more risks when being watched by women they find attractive.

(114) Pregnancy can increase a woman's libido.

(115) People who have sex
approximately three times
a week look several years
younger than those who don't.

(116) Experiencing 'butterflies of love'
sounds romantic, but in France
the phrase '*papillon d'amour*'
means having pubic lice.

 In several cities in Sweden, you
can get condoms delivered
to your home late at night.

118 The man who invented Kellogg's Corn Flakes was a zealous campaigner against masturbation, and believed a healthy diet would reduce sexual thoughts.

119 The average vagina is three to four inches long but can expand by 200 per cent when sexually aroused.

120 The more sex you have, the more you want.

121 The average American man's erect penis is five to seven inches long and four to six inches in circumference, according to The Kinsey Institute for Research in Sex, Gender, and Reproduction.

122 Abstaining from any sexual activity for three weeks makes testosterone levels peak and boosts the libido, creating the ultimate male orgasm.

Men have an average of
11 erections per day.

 The ancient Egyptians used
dried crocodile dung as a
contraceptive, as it contains
spermicidal properties.
They also used honey, and
condoms made of fabric.

 Men who are risk takers, easily
excited or have performance
anxiety have a higher likelihood
of cheating on their partner.

An Italian study in 1990 showed that people who have just fallen in love can share symptoms experienced by sufferers of Obsessive Compulsive Disorder (OCD).

 Erogenous zones swell with blood at the high point of sexual arousal, so areas such as the penis head or nipples can become hypersensitive during and after orgasm.

(128) In America, women's favoured style of underwear is bikini, followed by briefs, thongs, boy shorts and other styles; ten per cent of women occasionally wear no underwear to prevent visible panty lines (VPL).

(129) There are 500–1,000 deaths every year from autoerotic asphyxiation: self-strangulation to reduce blood to the brain for a more intense orgasm.

(130) The global research site OnePoll.com reported that women believe Spain, Brazil and Italy produce the best lovers. Englishmen were believed to be 'too lazy'.

(131) The most popular fetishes in the Western world are feet and shoes.

 Dendrophilia is a sexual attraction to trees.

Single women are more attracted to unavailable men than to single ones.

 Exercise improves blood flow and sexual response; female pro athletes have higher sexual satisfaction than women who don't exercise.

 Twelve per cent of adults claim to have had sex at work.

IN THE FIFTEENTH AND SIXTEENTH CENTURIES IT WAS HIGHLY FASHIONABLE FOR EUROPEAN MEN TO WEAR A CODPIECE – A FLAP OR POUCH THAT MEN WORE OVER THEIR TROUSERS TO EXAGGERATE THE SIZE OF THEIR MANHOOD.

Many Mongolian erotic paintings show sex scenes taking place on horseback.

 In the fifth century BC, something called an *olisbos*, which we would call a dildo, was sold in the port of Miletus in Greece.

 An erection requires an average of two tablespoons of blood.

(140) *The Art of Love* by the Greek courtesan Philaenis of Samos was written around the third century BC, with information on sex positions and aphrodisiacs. Although only fragments survive, it inspired the poet Ovid to create his own manual a few centuries later.

(141) The Roman poet Ovid's *The Art of Love* includes such advice for men as 'letting her miss you – but not for long', and for women 'trying young and older lovers'.

(142) Semen contains only one per cent sperm; the other fifty or so components include prolactin, oxytocin, serotonin and oestrone, all natural antidepressants, according to research published in *Scientific American*.

(143) Oscar Wilde's 1893 play *Salome* depicts probably the first striptease: the dance of the seven veils. This went on to become a standard in burlesque shows.

(144) Strippers earn more money when ovulating, probably because of sexually-stimulating pheromones they release at that stage of their menstrual cycles.

(145) An annual Masturbate-a-thon has been held in San Francisco at the Center for Sex and Culture since 2000 to make masturbating less taboo; the event raises money for sexual health. London hosted Europe's first Masturbate-a-thon on 5 August 2006.

146 The black widow spider not only eats her mate during or after sex; she can consume as many as 20 lovers in a day.

147 The sensitive area inside the vagina on the upper wall, the G-spot, is named after Dr Ernest Gräfenberg. In experiments in 1950, he found that attention to this area could trigger powerful orgasms and female ejaculation.

148

A SCOTTISH STUDY REVEALED THAT PEOPLE FOUND PUBLIC SPEAKING EASIER AFTER ORGASM.

The use of condoms in Nevada brothels is compulsory.

 Most women have one breast more sensitive than the other – often the left.

 Kissing burns approximately 2 calories per minute, or 120 calories per hour. The extra saliva released also helps clean the mouth, reducing the risk of tooth decay.

A poll found that 82 per cent of computer geeks claimed they put their partner's pleasure above their own (compared with only 41 per cent of fitness professionals doing so).

 The scent of vanilla – from a candle, cake or even ice cream – naturally boosts libido, making people feel calmer and less inhibited.

In Renaissance Europe, condoms were made of animal intestines or linen.

 Researchers found that 58 per cent of individuals who regularly use porn felt more comfortable with their sexuality and fulfilling their partner sexually.

 Thirty per cent of women aged 80 or over still have sexual intercourse.

157 Erectile dysfunction – or impotence – can be caused by stress, alcohol, smoking, diabetes or depression; it can be treated by therapy, medication or relaxing more.

158 The clitoris is comprised of around 8,000 nerve endings, making it the most sensitive and sensual part of the female anatomy. The tip of the penis has only around 4,000.

159 Researchers from The Kinsey Institute found that women today have less sex than their 1950s counterparts; we now 'live in an age where there is little unfilled leisure time'.

160 Alcohol is not an aphrodisiac but it reduces inhibition, relaxing people and increasing their confidence; it also opens small blood vessels, making people feel flushed and warm.

Oxytocin, one of the chemicals released in the body during sex, reduces pain by about 50 per cent.

 In Losevo near St Petersburg, Russia, the Bubble Baba Challenge takes place every year. This is a race in which people raft blow-up sex dolls on the Vuoksa River.

 Having sex at least once a week can improve immune function.

About 30 per cent of men
worldwide are circumcised. The
tip of an uncircumcised penis
is likely to be more sensitive
because it's not always exposed.

 'Shy nipples' are inverted –
just like 'innie' belly buttons.
It's normal and doesn't
affect stimulation.

 Syphilis was known as 'the
French Disease' in Italy and 'the
English Disease' in France.

Upon losing battles, apes have a habit of masturbating.

 Massaging the heel just under the ankle bone can increase sensation in a man's penis.

 Women who masturbate regularly are more likely to experience orgasm during sex with a partner.

170 Making a ring with your fingers and squeezing the base of the penis will prolong sex before orgasm.

171 In ancient Greece, the common slang for fellatio was 'playing the flute'.

172 A foetus can masturbate in the womb.

173 The longest erect human penis on record is 13.5 inches (34.29 cm) – but the owner said he found it difficult to get a girlfriend.

174 People who develop a sexual attraction towards buildings and other inanimate objects call themselves 'Objectum Sexuals'. One woman had a civil ceremony with the Eiffel Tower and changed her surname to Eiffel.

175 Pubic hair is intended to protect the genitals, and also to trap and hold 'sex scents', to enhance our partner's sexual arousal.

176 A 2012 study in Massachusetts found a link between high-fat diets and lower sperm counts.

177 Almost 53 per cent of women have used external stimulation such as sex toys.

Coffee, Tea or Me? is a 1967 account of the sexual exploits of two airline stewardesses, Trudy Baker and Rachel Jones. In 2002, the real author, Donald Bain, revealed the truth in his memoir.

 The word 'pornography' is derived from the Greek language, meaning 'the writing of prostitutes'.

 The smallest erect human penis on record was 1 cm long.

According to manufacturers, only six per cent of men use extra-large condoms.

 In Tremonton, Utah, it's illegal for a woman to have sex with a man while riding in an ambulance.

 When ovulating, women are more tolerant of chat-up lines and find high-testosterone men more attractive than at other stages of their cycle.

(184)

A RESEARCHER FOUND, WHEN INTERVIEWING HUNDREDS OF STRIPPERS, THAT '80 PER CENT OF THE JOB IS TALKING'.

In 2012, the manager of the Lake District's Damson Dene Hotel replaced the Bibles in guest rooms with copies of erotic bestseller *Fifty Shades of Grey*.

 A shaved pubic area is more likely to spread a sexually transmitted infection.

 Women are more likely to be sexually aroused when ovulating.

(188) In ancient China, drinking mercury or lead after sex was believed to prevent pregnancy; unfortunately, it often resulted in sterility or death.

(189) In Victorian times, a prostitute was known as a 'blowsy', and 'blow' was slang for ejaculation. By the 1930s, the act of fellatio was known as a blow job.

(190) The average 200-lb gorilla has a two-inch long penis.

191 Scientific studies have found that men with mild facial scars were more attractive to women than those without; but that the women didn't consider them marriage material.

192 The juice of the silphium plant was a popular contraceptive in ancient Rome. It became extinct by the end of the first century AD.

193 Kissing is more hygienic than shaking hands.

(194) A *Cosmopolitan* magazine survey found that foreplay between the average married couple tends to last 14–17 minutes, and the man reaches orgasm after 6 minutes of intercourse.

(195) The Aztecs had several sex goddesses, including Tlazolteotl, goddess of lust and sexual misdeeds; Tlaco, goddess of sexual longing; and Teicu, goddess of sexual appetite.

Having at least four orgasms a week can reduce a man's chances of getting prostate cancer.

 The average duration of sexual intercourse between minks is eight hours.

 The *Kama Sutra* states that a ram's or goat's testicle boiled in sweetened milk can stimulate sexual desire.

199

WOMEN WITH A PHD
ARE TWICE AS LIKELY
TO BE INTERESTED IN
A ONE-NIGHT STAND
AS THOSE WITH A
BACHELOR'S DEGREE.

(200) The National Institute of Business Management in New York notes that one in every ten secretaries admits to having a romantic involvement with her boss; only a quarter report it having an adverse effect on their career.

(201) In Harrisburg, Pennsylvania, it is illegal to have sex with a truck driver in a tollbooth.

Only one per cent of women can achieve orgasm from breast stimulation alone.

 A survey conducted by condom manufacturer Durex found that of all nations, Austrians engage in the most oral sex.

 Condoms that make the penis less sensitive can help prevent premature ejaculation.

A woman is more likely to orgasm when the walls of her vagina are stimulated by a thicker penis.

 A man needs anything from two minutes to two weeks to regain an erection.

 Vorarephilia is a sexual attraction to eating, or being eaten by, others.

As surgery can cause nerve damage, some women with breast implants report a loss of sensitivity, while others claim they derive increased sexual pleasure from having new breasts.

 In seventeenth-century Spain, a woman could expose her breasts, but feet were considered sexual and it was illegal for anyone other than a woman's husband to see her bare feet.

210   The ancient Romans would crush a first-time rapist's gonads between two stones as punishment for his crime.

211   In Brazil, people have sex for an average of 30 minutes – compared to ten minutes in Thailand.

212   A study of 900 films over a four-year period found that scenes including sex and nudity did not increase a film's success.

213 'Glans condoms' – caps covering the head of the penis – were used in Asia before the fifteenth century and could be made of oiled silk paper, lamb intestines, tortoise shell or animal horn.

214 A 2008 study found that having an orgasm can cure a blocked nose; sex acts as a natural antihistamine, and can also help with asthma and hay fever.

(215)

CERTAIN FEMALE PENGUINS WILL OFFER SEXUAL FAVOURS TO SINGLE MALES IN EXCHANGE FOR PEBBLES TO BUILD THEIR NESTS.

216 It's illegal to have sex on a motorbike in London.

217 During the Great Depression in America, 'Tijuana bibles' were a popular form of entertainment: cheap stapled comics containing erotic stories.

218 Hugh Hefner published the first edition of *Playboy* Magazine in America in December 1953; a nude Marilyn Monroe was the first *Playboy* centrefold.

219 In 1524, Marcantonio Raimondi published 16 engravings of characters from classical history having sex – and was sent to prison for a year by the Pope. His official crime was copyright violation, but the pornographic content was no doubt the real issue.

220 According to one study, swallowing her partner's semen can lower a woman's blood pressure and lower her risks of getting pre-eclampsia.

(221) As well as the genitals and the breasts, the inner nose also swells during intercourse – this is because it is made from the same type of erectile tissue as the penis.

(222) Men are biologically attracted to breasts, but not only large breasts: body proportions and distribution of body fat are more important than breast size.

223 The Aztecs believed that the avocado was a powerful aphrodisiac, and the fruit carried a sexual stigma until the nineteenth century, when growers campaigned to make it more acceptable to consumers.

224 Sixteenth-century Canadians used home-brewed alcohol with dried beaver testicles ground up into a fine powder as an aphrodisiac.

According to a survey of sex shop owners, the most popular flavour for edible underwear is cherry, and the least popular is chocolate.

 Scientific studies have shown that heterosexual men who looked at porn of two men and one woman produced more sperm than those who looked at just women, perhaps because seeing competition makes the man increase his chances at impregnating a female.

The symbols used for male and female represent Mars and Venus – a shield and spear for the male, and a hand mirror for the female.

 In medieval Europe, weasel testicles were believed to prevent pregnancy.

The word 'sexennial' has nothing to do with sex; it means 'occurring every six years', which we hope doesn't describe sex.

 Researchers claim that a woman who wears white cotton knickers tends to be a low-maintenance partner.

 Most male giraffes are bisexual.

A head massage helps release oxytocin, a hormone that provides a sense of calm while enhancing sexual pleasure.

 Opposites attract because biologically we seek out potential mates with different DNA.

 In Italy, red underwear is considered to be lucky.

235

PEACHES, BANANAS, PINE NUTS, MUSSELS, EELS, HORSERADISH, ASPARAGUS, CUCUMBERS, AND ONIONS ARE ALL BELIEVED TO HAVE APHRODISIAC QUALITIES.

Aphrodisiacs are named after Aphrodite, the Greek goddess of love, pleasure and procreation.

 Truffles, caviar, strawberries, oysters and chocolate are also well known as being conducive to love.

 According to *Playboy*, more Americans lose their virginity in June than any other month.

Except for a pair of Cohan gorillas, bonobos are the only non-humans to have been observed engaged in face-to-face sex, kissing with tongues and oral sex.

 When bonobos find a new feeding ground, the excitement will usually lead to communal sexual activity.

 A man's penis shrinks temporarily when his favourite football team scores.

Am Abend, or *In the Evening*, is one of the earliest pornographic films, produced in Germany in 1910. It starts with voyeurism, as a man watches a woman masturbating in her bedroom.

 Cervical caps made of gold or silver were once the most fashionable form of contraception – before science discovered Toxic Shock Syndrome.

If you're a member of the Nevada legislature, you cannot conduct business, while in session, wearing a penis costume.

 In Santa Cruz, Bolivia, it is illegal for a man to have sex with a woman and her daughter at the same time.

A MAN CAN INCREASE HIS TESTOSTERONE LEVELS BY UP TO 30 PER CENT – AND THEREFORE IMPROVE HIS LIBIDO – BY PLAYING FOOTBALL.

The colour red is a turn-on: both men and women who wear red are considered more attractive.

 A man's sweat glands release a hormone called androstadienone, which increases women's sexual arousal by up to 200 per cent.

 Reproduction without sex is called parthenogenesis.

250 Regular Pilates classes lead to better flexibility, more strength in the upper body and improved abdominal power – all good for trying different sex positions, which can make orgasms more intense.

251 The area of the male brain responsible for sexual pursuit is 2.5 times larger than the female equivalent, and it is fuelled by 10 to 15 times the amount of testosterone.

(252) In Anniston, Alabama, if a woman loses a game of pool, it is illegal for her to settle her tab with sex.

(253) Taiwanese women use vibrators more than the women of other nations.

(254) Although it may appear tiny, the clitoris is shaped like a wishbone and is about 7.5 to 11.5 cm long.

In 1837, there were over fifty pornographic shops on London's Holywell Street. This scurrilous address was lost when The Strand was widened in 1900.

 One of the first magazines to display photographs of the female nude was the French magazine *Le Frisson* at the turn of the twentieth century; French magazines commonly published nudes under the guise of naturism.

The *Kama Sutra* contains 529 sex positions, including eight different types of oral sex.

 In the Middle Ages people preferred small breasts and women wore corsets to flatten their chests.

 During the Renaissance it was popular in Spain to have cone-shaped breasts.

In mythology, Aphrodite was born when the god Cronus cut off Uranus' genitals and threw them in the sea.

 Psychotria elata, a plant that grows in Central and South American tropical forests, has a flower that resembles two luscious, bright-red lipsticked lips – hence its nickname, Hooker's Lips.

A couple are less likely to have sex problems if they make the bedroom a place to relax, and not argue or talk about serious issues.

 In AD 953, Princess Olga of Kiev introduced a law whereby men could return their wives if they found out they were not virgins, asking for monetary or material compensation.

264 Researchers found that women get physically aroused by a wider variety of erotic imagery than men do.

 265 Lesbians have lower rates of sexual diseases than any other sexually active adults.

 266 During a recession, the market for expensive sex-related entertainment, such as strip clubs and phone sex, plummets.

In 1919, before being elected President of America, Franklin Roosevelt is believed to have created a special undercover unit in the Navy to entrap gay men by performing oral sex on suspected homosexuals.

 A study found that higher rates of poverty lead to more sex – except when couples are concerned about the cost of getting pregnant.

269

A MAN'S BEARD GROWS FASTEST WHEN HE ANTICIPATES SEX.

Almost a third of respondents in a survey said they were masturbating more since the recent UK recession began.

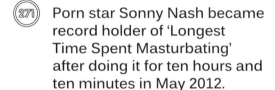 Porn star Sonny Nash became record holder of 'Longest Time Spent Masturbating' after doing it for ten hours and ten minutes in May 2012.

 An erect giraffe penis is four feet long.

273 Male honeybees only have sex once in their lives, because the act of mating causes the penis and associated abdominal tissues to be ripped from their body, killing them.

274 Sperm in a sperm bank is kept at −196.111 °C and will last indefinitely at that temperature.

275 In Newcastle, Wyoming, it is illegal to have sex inside a store's walk-in meat freezer.

People who are critical and judgemental of others are less likely to be open-minded when it comes to sex.

 Researchers at the University of California found that it takes the male brain only a fifth of a second to decide if a woman is sexually attractive or not – causing the man's pupils to dilate, his testosterone to surge, and his heart rate to accelerate.

The term 'gigolo' is now used for a male prostitute, but in the 1920s it meant a dancing partner and companion, kept by a woman.

 In some parts of the world, animal species such as rhinos, tigers and bears have become endangered because their horns or private parts are used as aphrodisiacs, although they have no real effect.

According to medical literature, there have been approximately 80 cases of a man being born with two penises.

 Plant-based substances such as ginseng or vanilla, patchouli or musk scents are believed to stimulate sexual energy.

According to the journal *Cephalalgia*, regular sex can alleviate migraines.

283

THOSE WHO ORGASM
TWICE A WEEK CAN
ADD UP TO EIGHT
YEARS TO THEIR LIFE,
ACCORDING TO A 1997
STUDY IN THE *BRITISH
MEDICAL JOURNAL.*

Good listeners are often good in bed. Someone who is engaged by your conversation and alert to conversational cues is more likely to be responsive to sexual needs.

 According to ancient Jewish law, labourers were advised to have intercourse with their wives twice a week; ass drivers only once a week.

The A-spot, or anterior fornix, is on the upper wall of the vagina near the cervix and arousing it leads to pleasure and lubrication.

 Male goats urinate on themselves to attract females.

 As protection against HIV, condoms make sex 10,000 times safer than unprotected sex.

Sex is good for the immune system, heart and brain.

 The vagina is a self-cleaning organ, like the eye.

 On 16 February 1899, the President of France, Félix Faure, died in his office at the Élysée Palace while engaging in sexual activities.

The Kinsey Report: Sexual Behaviour in the Human Female, published in 1953, claimed that 15 per cent of women were capable of multiple orgasms.

 There are latex-free condoms made of polyurethane and polyisoprene for people with latex allergies.

 Lions can mate up to 50 times a day.

295 If a potential partner shows deep enthusiasm for their work or hobby, it may be a good sign that they will be able to stay excited and focused for passionate sex.

296 'Morning dew' is a slang term for vaginal lubrication, or sexual arousal, on waking up. 'Morning wood' is the male equivalent.

297

SOME SLANG FOR SEX:
A BIT OF HOW'S YOUR
FATHER; BONK; DO THE
HORIZONTAL BOP; GET
DOWN AND DIRTY; GIVE
IT UP; HIT A HOME RUN;
TAKE OLD ONE-EYE TO
THE OPTOMETRIST.

(298) The word 'vagina' means 'sheath' or 'scabbard' in Latin, suggesting that sexual activity and warfare have been connected for thousands of years.

(299) In AD 401, St Augustine wrote, 'Nothing is so powerful in drawing the spirit of a man downwards as the caresses of a woman.'

In Oxford, Ohio, it's illegal for a woman to strip off her clothing while standing in front of a picture of a man.

 Male bats have the highest rate of homosexuality of any mammal.

 The highest number of large-cup bras are sold in the UK; Japan usually sells most of the smallest cup sizes.

ITHYPHALLOPHOBICS ARE AFRAID OF SEEING OR HAVING AN ERECT PENIS.

On a biological level, men have evolved to focus on the features of a woman that suggest fertility – large breasts, a small waist and full hips indicate that a woman is young, healthy and probably not already pregnant.

 At least half of all sexually active men and women will have a genital HPV (human papillomavirus) during their lives; in 90 per cent of cases, the body's immune system will fight off the disease in two years.

A recent study of 2,000 Brits revealed that people with caramel-coloured bedrooms get the most sex: on average, three times per week.

 Women will receive twice as many responses to their profile page on an Internet dating site if they use a photo.

The way a man stands can contribute up to 80 per cent of a woman's first impression of him.

 Women fantasise more during sex to increase sexual pleasure than men do.

 On average, men lose their virginity aged 16.9; women at a slightly older 17.4.

311　Sitophiliacs are sexually aroused by food – by eating it or touching it.

312　Too much caffeine can overstimulate the adrenal glands, producing stress hormones that have a negative impact on libido.

313　A cup of coffee can provide energy and stamina for sex.

314 Professor Arthur Arun, a New York psychologist, discovered that if two strangers share personal information and stare deeply into each other's eyes, they are highly likely to be attracted to each other.

315 The ancient Greek god of fertility, Priapus, is often shown with a disproportionately large erection. His statue was often used to protect property boundaries, and travellers would stroke the penis as they passed by.

(316) Lying down can reduce sensitivity to sound and smell, which could explain why other positions offer more sexual thrills.

(317) Men can achieve multiple orgasms, but the first must happen without ejaculation.

(318) In Uganda, some women apply a herb mixture to their labia to elongate them and attract men.

Commercial cold and flu remedies can reduce libido, as can antihistamines and blood pressure pills.

 The bleach-like smell of semen comes from the natural chemical spermine that protects sperm from vaginal acids.

 Sex triggers brain chemicals that can improve creativity.

322 Masturbation and coitus interruptus are both sometimes referred to as 'onanism', thanks to the Biblical story of Onan, who 'spilled his seed' deliberately on the ground.

323 People fall asleep after orgasm because it triggers the parasympathetic nervous system, activating the body's 'rest and digest' function.

Priapism is a medical condition, sometimes painful, where the erection persists for several hours.

 The top five countries with the lowest recorded average age for having sex for the first time are Iceland (where the age is 15.6 years), Denmark, Sweden, Finland and Norway. The country with the highest recorded average age is Malaysia (23 years).

The Lake Duck has the longest penis, in relation to body-length, of all vertebrates.

 Eating chilli, curry, or any other hot spice can act like an aphrodisiac by increasing heart rate and causing us to perspire.

 Jacques de Béthencourt was a sixteenth-century French physician famous for coining the term 'venereal disease'.

329 In a 1995 study in Switzerland, women were asked to sniff sweaty T-shirts. They consistently preferred the smell of men whose immune systems were different from their own.

330 Overweight men have higher levels of the female estradiol hormone, blocking male hormones and delaying orgasm: heavier men are able to make love for longer.

331 Going on a date night with your partner is known to boost the libido.

332 Men whose index and ring fingers are mismatched are likelier to have higher than average levels of testosterone.

333 Snakes and lizards have two penises, though they only use one during mating.

MATING SNAILS STAB
THEIR PARTNERS
WITH LOVE DARTS –
POSSIBLY TO MAKE THEM
SLOWER TO RE-MATE.

People who have just fallen
in love have high levels of the
neurotransmitter dopamine
in their brains. This creates a
pleasure rush similar to cocaine!

 When prairie voles mate,
their brain chemistry changes
permanently, and they form
a strong pair-bond that lasts
for the rest of their lives.

Women who cycle 100 miles a week have been found to experience decreased sexual sensation.

 While mating underwater for long periods, the male sea snake can only come up for air when the female swims to the surface.

 In Moroccan mythology, Qandisa is the goddess of lust who seduces men before driving them insane.

A larger area of the male brain is designated for sex, compared to the female brain, and researchers have found that the chemicals testosterone and oestrogen stop men thinking about long-term consequences of their actions.

 A 2011 study found that young men think about sleep and food as often as they think about sex.

Wearing high heels may strengthen the pelvic muscles, which helps orgasm. In ancient Rome, only prostitutes were allowed to wear high heels.

 Women may find they orgasm more just before or during their period: more blood flow in the pelvis and natural lubrication leads to increased pleasure.

 Canadian porcupines kiss one another on the lips.

In eighteenth- and nineteenth-century Italy, a *cicisbeo* or *cavalier servente* was the lover of a married woman.

 In Connorsville, Wisconsin, it's illegal for a man to shoot a gun when his female partner has an orgasm.

 A man's testicles increase in size when he's sexually excited.

Aristophanes, the fifth-century BC Greek comedy playwright, devised 106 ways of describing the male genitals and 91 for those of the female.

 In ancient Greece, there was an annual procession for Dionysus, when the men carried a large phallus; the city of Tyrnavos in Greece still holds an annual phallus festival during Lent. Similar parades in Japan are known as Kanamara Matsuri.

In Idaho, couples are not allowed to engage in any public display of affection for more than 18 minutes.

 The science writer, Mary Roach and her husband became the first people to be filmed having sex in 4D, in 2008.

 Cosmopolitan magazine says that, according to its readers, 32 per cent have lied about how many people they've slept with.

Taco Bell's 'Chilito' changed its name to the 'Chili Cheese Burrito' when it was discovered that *chilito* in Spanish means 'small penis'.

 According to scientists, it takes between 30 seconds and four minutes to decide if you fancy somebody.

Breast size is mostly hereditary but also affected by age, diet, pregnancy, menstruation and body weight.

 In the nineteenth century, you could purchase a guidebook to the brothels of London and New York.

 A pair of male homosexual penguins at Central Park Zoo adopted and raised a baby penguin together in 2003.

358) The fertility of female pigs
being artificially inseminated is
improved if they are stimulated
to orgasm during the process.
Special pig vibrators are
available to help those who
prefer not to do this by hand.

359) In a survey, more than a fifth
of people around the world
would rather go out with
their friends than have sex.
Ten per cent would rather
play sport or go shopping.

Non-lubricated condoms
are distributed among the
armed forces as emergency
water holders; they hold
about a gallon of water.

 When a man is separated
from his sexual partner, his
sperm count decreases.

 Sex can temporarily alleviate
mild depression by releasing
endorphins into the blood,
creating a feeling of well-being.

A study found that heterosexual women can be turned on just as much by watching female-only erotica as they can by watching sex between men and women.

 An ancient law in Alabama bans men from attempting to seduce 'a chaste woman by means of temptation, arts, deception, flattery or a promise of marriage'.

365 The name of the Wyoming mountain range Grand Tetons means 'Big Teats' in French, though some also claim the name comes from the Teton Sioux tribe of Native Americans.

366 A University of Leeds study found that a stripper typically earns about the same as an American attorney or computer programmer, and that strippers have high levels of job satisfaction.

Orgasms can cause women to have bad breath, but it only lasts for around an hour after intercourse.

 Research in 2010 found that women who feel confident about how their private parts look find it easier to orgasm.

 Men and women are equally likely to dream about sex, and both can have orgasms while sleeping.

If you're interested in finding out
more about our books,
find us on Facebook at
Summersdale Publishers
and follow us on Twitter at
@Summersdale.

www.summersdale.com

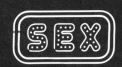

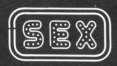